Paleo Smoothies

Super Delicious & Filling, Protein-Packed, Low in Sugar, Gluten-Free, Easy to Make, Fruit and Veggie SUPERFOOD Smoothie RECIPES for Natural Weight Loss and Unstoppable Energy

By Elena Garcia

Copyright Elena Garcia © 2019

All rights reserved. No part of this publication may be reproduced, stored in a retrieval system, or transmitted, in any form or by any means, electronic, mechanical, photocopying, recording or otherwise, without the prior written permission of the author and the publishers.

The scanning, uploading, and distribution of this book via the Internet or via any other means without the permission of the author is illegal and punishable by law. Please purchase only authorized electronic editions, and do not participate in or encourage electronic piracy of copyrighted materials.

Disclaimer

A physician has not written the information in this book. It is advisable that you visit a qualified dietician so that you can obtain a highly personalized treatment for your case, especially if you want to lose weight effectively. This book is for informational and educational purposes only and is not intended for medical purposes. Please consult your physician before making any drastic changes to your diet.

All information in this book has been carefully researched and checked for factual accuracy. However, the author and publishers make no warranty, expressed or implied, that the information contained herein is appropriate for every individual, situation or purpose, and assume no responsibility for errors or omission. The reader assumes the risk and full responsibility for all actions and the author will not be held liable for any loss or damage, whether consequential, incidental, and special or otherwise, that may result from the information presented in this publication.

The book is not intended to provide medical advice or to take the place of medical advice and treatment from your personal physician. Readers are advised to consult their own doctors or other qualified health professionals regarding the treatment of medical conditions. The author shall not be held liable or responsible for any misunderstanding or misuse of the information contained in this book. The information is not intended to diagnose, treat or cure any disease.

Why Paleo Smoothie Recipes?................................8

Paleo Smoothies – Easy Guidelines and Templates.......12

Recipe Measurements 14

Sexy Paleo Smoothie Recipes 15

    Recipe #1 Banana Dream Treat Smoothie 16

    Recipe #2 Berry Green Healer 17

    Recipe #3 Paleo Healthy Fat & Protein Smoothie.......18

    Recipe #4 Sexy Veggie Blend......................................19

    Recipe #5 Simple Snack Smoothie..............................20

    Recipe #6 Healing Green Energy 21

    Recipe #7 Work Better Smoothie 22

    Recipe #8 Easy Weight Loss Smoothie 23

    Recipe #9 Mango Papaya Madness............................24

    Recipe #10 Sweet Guilt Free Smoothie 25

    Recipe #11 Veggie Freak 26

    Recipe #12 Creamy Dream Smoothie 27

    Recipe #13 Mango Protein Smoothie........................28

    Recipe #14 Easy Tropical Smoothie 29

    Recipe #15 Cucumber Paleo Soup Smoothie 30

    Recipe #16 Paleo Zucchini Dream 31

    Recipe #17 Watermelon Hydration 32

    Recipe #18 Mediterranean Gazpacho Smoothness 33

Recipe #19 Celery Veggie Snack.................................... 34

Recipe #20 Kale Weight Loss Magician 35

Recipe #21 Easy Tahini Smoothie 36

Recipe #22 Full Brain Power 37

Recipe #23 Good Carbs Smoothie............................... 38

Recipe #24 Green Date Smoothie 39

Recipe #25 Easy Berry Best.. 40

Recipe #26 Watermelon Refreshment 41

Recipe #27 Papaya Weight Loss Smoothie Tea 42

Recipe #28 Creamy Balancer 43

Recipe #29 Vitamin C Delight 44

Recipe #30 Creamy Spinach Beauty Smoothie 45

Recipe 31 Green Refreshment 46

Recipe #32 Beautiful Skin Smoothie 47

Recipe #33 Creamy Paleo Protein Smoothie 48

Recipe #34 Ginger Mystery Smoothie........................ 49

Recipe #35 Tasty Veggie Smoothie 50

Recipe #36 Spicy Spinach Smoothie........................... 51

Recipe #37 Easy Antioxidant Smoothie...................... 52

Recipe #38 Simple Apple Lemon Juice 53

Recipe #39 Honeydew Melon Green Juice 54

Recipe #40 Easy Green Protein Smoothie 55

Recipe #41 Green Coconut Smoothie 56

Recipe #42 Hidden Broccoli Smoothie 57

Recipe #43 Green Tea Fat Burn Smoothie 58

Recipe #44 Healthy Glow Smoothie 59

Recipe #45 Antioxidant Veggie Smoothie 60

Recipe #46 Easy Beet Smoothie 61

Recipe #47 Simple Nutrition Smoothie 62

Recipe #48 Arugula Power Olive Smoothie 63

Recipe #49 Tantalizing Green Smoothie Soup 64

Recipe #50 Re-Balancing Carrot Smoothie 65

Recipe #51 Easy Almond Butter & Banana Smoothie . 66

Recipe #52 Sexy Flaxseed Smoothie 67

Recipe #53 Blueberry Optimal Protein Smoothie 68

Recipe #54 Mango & Almond Butter Smoothie 70

Recipe #55 Cinnamon Protein Smoothie 71

Recipe #56 Spinach & Avocado Smoothie 72

Recipe #57 The Green Machine Protein Smoothie 73

Recipe #57 Goji Berry Dream Smoothie 74

Recipe #58 Paleo Chocolate Smoothie 76

Recipe # 59 Chia Coconut Smoothie 77

Recipe #60 Pumpkin Seed Protein Smoothie 78

Final Words and Your Paleo Quick Start Guide 80

Paleo Lifestyle Made Easy 80

More Books in the Paleo – Healthy Lifestyle Series 90

PALEO SMOOTHIES - INTRODUCTION

Why Paleo Smoothie Recipes?

Are you looking for easy to follow healthy recipes to help you look and feel amazing?

Sick and tired of spending long hours in your kitchen trying to figure out how to put some healthy meals together?

Or maybe you tried something healthy, but it didn't taste good and you lost your motivation?

What about some easy, take-away meals?
Or quick snack and breakfast ideas?

Whatever your health and fitness goal is, you will find your answers in Paleo Smoothies.

Paleo Smoothies offer the most effective, fruit, veggie and superfood blends that are:

-low in sugar

-rich in natural protein (all Paleo approved), both plant-based protein and animal protein

-all gluten-free

-full of antioxidants

-super filling

PALEO SMOOTHIES - INTRODUCTION

Paleo smoothies are tasty, easy and quick to prepare even on a busy schedule. They can be used as a quick snack or breakfast. These smoothies are great for weight loss being full of fiber, vitamins and minerals. Some people find them useful for fasting or as a meal replacement.

While salads are great and super healthy, they are much more time-consuming than smoothies. To make a smoothie, you just throw it all into a blender, and you don't need to worry about artistically cutting all the ingredients. Not at all. Oh, and it only takes a few minutes to drink a smoothie, or quickly go through a thick-a-la-soup smoothie.

But with salads? OMG. It will definitely take longer.

(I love salads as well, and following that passion I have even written a book called Paleo Salads. But, smoothies are much easier than salads. Especially, if you are on a super busy schedule, and want to give your mouth and digestive system a rest).

As far as time and preparation are concerned, smoothies also beat juicing. Extracting the juices from fruits and veggies takes much longer than just blending it all, and there is always more clean-up involved with juicing. Yea, I love juicing too, and I set up my juicer like twice a week, to do some massive batch juicing. I do it for my health, but very often I find myself much more motivated to do smoothies instead.

Oh, and smoothies are less expensive than juicing. Trust me on that one!

PALEO SMOOTHIES - INTRODUCTION

So, how do you go about creating super healthy paleo smoothies that you enjoy and that can also help you with weight loss while improving your energy levels?

The best part is- you don't need to be a great cook. Not at all. And you can get super creative and even if you don't follow the recipes 100%, you are still bound to come up with something amazing.

You can play around with many of the ingredients and come up with your own favorites. You can leave things out or add some new ones so that you create the taste you love. That's what I love about Paleo Smoothies, they are so changeable but still so tasty and nutritious. Change things up and try something new. Have fun, be creative!

What I really love about Paleo fruit smoothies is that they can be an amazing guilt-free, dairy-free treat and be turned into an ice-cream as well. Many "fruity" Paleo smoothies also sneak in some greens and veggies, which makes them excellent, beginner friendly smoothies.

Veggie Paleo smoothies, on the other hand, can be turned into a delicious soup. You can even spice it up with many oriental herbs, chili and some meat or fish leftovers. That will allow you to spend less time in the kitchen, and save your time and money on mindless cooking or eating out.

It's so ridiculously easy…you just blend some ingredients following the recipe and add in some paleo friendly foods like nuts, seeds,

PALEO SMOOTHIES - INTRODUCTION

meat, seafood, hard-boiled eggs, olives...and voila- you have a delicious, satisfying meal within a few minutes. And you get rid of some leftovers in a creative way.

In case you are new to a Paleo diet or healthy eating, don't worry. At the end of this guide, you will find some easy to follow instructions to help you kickstart your journey.

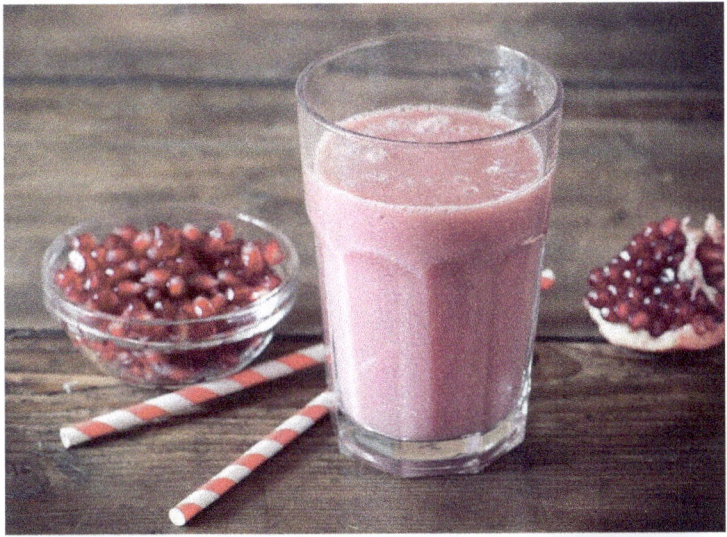

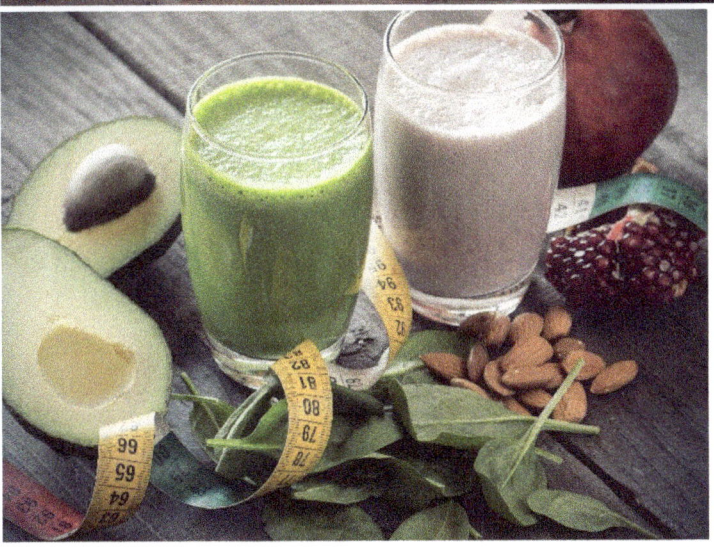

Paleo Smoothies – Easy Guidelines and "Templates"

You are probably wondering what ingredients you need to get started on making paleo smoothies.

It's very simple. You need:

-fresh fruits

-fresh veggies

-fresh greens of your choice

-paleo friendly, non-dairy, soy-free milk or yoghurt, for example: almond, coconut, hazelnut, cashew...

-you can also use coconut water, filtered water, ice cubes, or even herbal infusions (you will see how to go about it when you dive into the recipes)

-nuts, seeds, non-dairy plant-based protein, for example: chia seeds, almonds, cashews

-some green powders, like for example: spirulina

-good oils, for example coconut oil, avocado oil, olive oil

-herbs and spices, for example cinnamon powder, rosemary, curry, chilly (depends on a smoothie of course, some smoothies will be sweet, and some will be sour or spicy)
Also, feel free to experiment. Nothing is set in stone.
You can use our recipes to create your own.
The most important thing is to <u>listen to your body</u>.

You can always skip an ingredient you don't like, or replace it with something similar.

For example, coconut milk can be replaced with almond milk, or cashew milk, or any other plant based non-dairy milk of your choice.

This approach will give you more creativity and it will also release the stress. Making smoothies should be exciting and fun!

Final Note: be sure to wash all the fruits and veggies before turning them into smoothies. Also, try to go for fresh, local produce.

You can always make a big smoothie and store it in a fridge (to have it within the next 24 hours to get the most out of it).
In fact, I am a big fan of "batch-blending".

That way, you can save even more time and energy.

Now, without any further ado, let's get into the Paleo smoothie recipes!

Recipe Measurements

The cup measurement I use is the American Cup measurement.

I also use it for dry ingredients. If you are new to it, let me help you:

If you don't have American Cup measures, just use a metric or imperial liquid measuring jug and fill your jug with your ingredient to the corresponding level. Here's how to go about it:

1 American Cup= 250ml= 8 fl.oz.

For example:

If a recipe calls for 1 cup of almonds, simply place your almonds into your measuring jug until it reaches the 250 ml/8oz mark.

I hope you found it helpful. I know that different countries use different measurements and I wanted to make things simple for you. I have also noticed that very often those who are used to American Cup measurements complain about metric measurements and vice versa. However, if you apply what I have just explained, you will find it easy to use both.

Sexy Paleo Smoothie Recipes

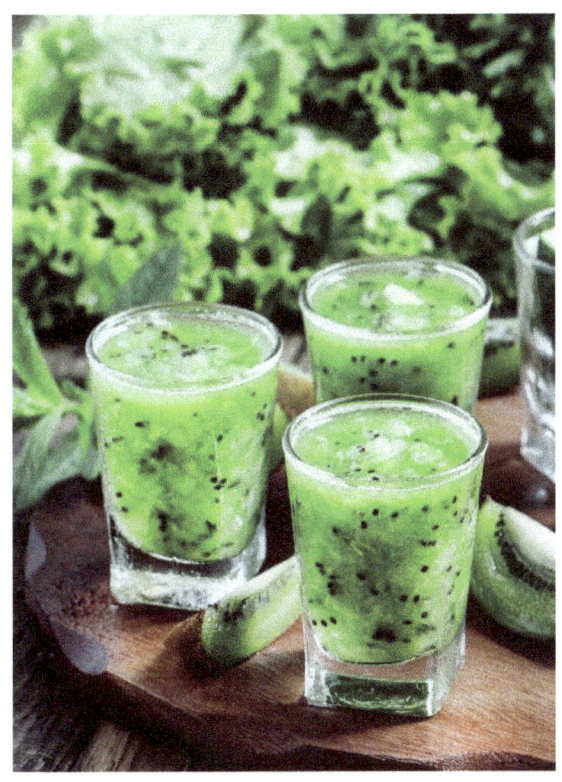

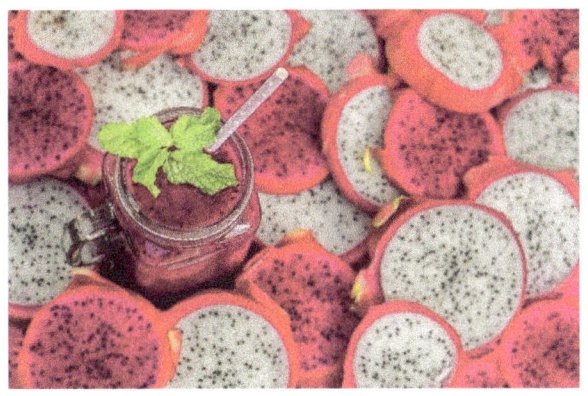

DELICIOUS PALEO SMOOTHIE RECIPES

Recipe #1 Banana Dream Treat Smoothie

This banana smoothie uses spirulina and kale, helping you to get in some extra nutrients in. It offers a fantastic energy boost that will help you prevent sugar cravings.

Serves 1-2

Ingredients:
- 1 big apple, peeled
- 1 small banana, peeled
- 1 tablespoon Spirulina
- 1 tablespoon chia seeds or chia seed powder
- Half cup kale, peeled
- 1 cup almond milk
- A few ice cubes

Instructions:
1. Place all the above ingredients in your blender.
2. Blend well.
3. Serve and enjoy!

DELICIOUS PALEO SMOOTHIE RECIPES

Recipe #2 Berry Green Healer

Coconut water is totally optional in this recipe. You can also use any Paleo friendly, nut milk of your choice or filtered water. However, coconut water is a great addition as it makes this smoothie much more refreshing and adds in more nutrients. Personally, I love this smoothie after my workouts or on a hot summer day.

Serves: 2
Ingredients:
- 1.5 cup of coconut water, or "normal", filtered water, or any paleo friendly, dairy-free nut milk of your choice
- 1 cup blueberries
- 1 cup baby spinach, washed
- 2 tablespoons raw organic honey
- 1 teaspoon cinnamon powder (yummy, it really makes it taste so good and is an aphrodisiac)
- Half cup ice

Instructions:
1. Put all ingredients in a blender.
2. Pulse to desired consistency.
3. Enjoy!

DELICIOUS PALEO SMOOTHIE RECIPES

Recipe #3 Paleo Healthy Fat & Protein Smoothie

Egg yolks are a great addition to any smoothie on the paleo plan. Make sure they are organic and free-range or pasture raised. We are also adding in some good fats to make sure you feel energized throughout the day.

Serves: 1
Ingredients:
- 1 small avocado, peeled and pitted
- 1 large cucumber, peeled and pitted
- 2 cups of coconut or almond milk
- A few leaves of kale
- half cup of fresh spinach
- 2 egg yolks, organic
- Himalayan salt and black pepper to taste

Instructions:
1. In a blender, add all the above ingredients except for the ice. Blend well.
2. Add ice and pulse until smooth.
3. Enjoy!

Recipe #4 Sexy Veggie Blend

You know veggies are good for you. But how to make sure you get your daily portion of veggies quickly and almost effortlessly? This smoothie recipe might be the answer you have been searching for.

Serves: 2-3

Ingredients:
- 2 big carrots, peeled and chopped
- 2 stalks celery, chopped
- 1 cucumber, peeled and chopped
- 1 zucchini, peeled and chopped
- 1 lemon, peeled
- 1 beetroot, peeled
- 1 big red bell pepper, peeled and chopped
- 2 cups almond milk, or any other paleo nut milk of your choice
- Optional: 1 tablespoon chia seeds or any paleo friendly, dairy-free protein powder of your choice

Instructions:
1. Blend all and pulse in ice.
2. Enjoy!

Recipe #5 Simple Snack Smoothie

Cranberries are high in vitamin C, among many other antioxidants. They help the body's conversion of glucose to energy.
Combined with other ingredients and healthy fats and protein, they will help you stay energized for hours.

Serves: 2

Ingredients:
- 2 teaspoons organic avocado oil
- 2 organic free-range egg yolks
- Handful of spinach, washed
- 1 small banana, peeled
- Half cup cranberries
- 1 cup coconut milk
- Ice cubes

Instructions:
1. Blend all and pulse in some ice if needed.
2. Enjoy!

Recipe #6 Healing Green Energy

Feeling fatigued? The best way to beat fatigue naturally is by adding more greens and green smoothies to your diet. They are rich in alkaline minerals such as Magnesium and Potassium. Chlorophyll, naturally present in greens, is full of vitamins and anti-oxidants to help you get rid of toxins and feel energized all day long. Spinach is rich in Iron. Oranges spice it up with natural Vitamin C to help your body absorb that iron faster.

Serves: 3
Ingredients:
- Half cup broccoli florets, cooked and chopped
- 1 cup spinach
- 1 egg yolk
- 1 tablespoon almond butter
- 1 tablespoon coconut oil
- Handful of pepitas
- 1 apple peeled and chopped
- 1 orange, peeled
- 1 cup coconut water
- A few ice cubes

Instructions:
1. Blend all the above ingredients together.
2. Enjoy!

Recipe #7 Work Better Smoothie

This smoothie is perfect if you need to study, work or concentrate for long periods of time. It offers a healing blend of blueberries (full of anti-oxidants), good fats from avocado, healthy protein from nut milk as well as healing chlorophyll from greens.

Serves: 2

Ingredients:
- 1 cup blueberries, fresh
- 1 avocado, peeled and pitted
- 1 cup of almond or cashew or almond milk
- Half cup arugula leaves
- A few dates, pitted
- One lime, peeled

Instructions:
1. Place all the above ingredients in a blender, mix well and enjoy!

Recipe #8 Easy Weight Loss Smoothie

This smoothie is rich in Vitamins and minerals, very hydrating, low in calories as well as high in protein and low in carbs. Perfect to stimulate natural weight loss, without going hungry or feeling deprived.

Serves: 3-4
Ingredients:
- 1 cup of blueberries, fresh
- 1 cup raspberries, fresh
- 1 cup coconut water
- 1 grapefruit, peeled
- A handful of almonds (soaked)
- 1 tablespoon chia seeds or chia seed powder
- 1 teaspoon spirulina powder

Instructions:
1. Blend all.
2. Serve and Enjoy!

Recipe #9 Mango Papaya Madness

This simple recipe combines the sweetness of mangos with the healing, alkalizing properties of spinach. Raw honey helps maintain a healthy immune system and papaya helps digestion.

Serves: 2-3
Ingredients:
- 1 cup mango, peeled and chopped
- 1 cup papaya, peeled and chopped
- 1 cup filtered water, or any herbal infusion of your choice (for example: mint)
- Half cup spinach
- 1 tablespoon raw honey
- A few ice cubes (optional)

Instructions:
1. Add all the above ingredients in a blender and blend well.
2. Pour and enjoy!

Recipe #10 Sweet Guilt Free Smoothie

The cinnamon in this smoothie helps to regulate blood sugar and insulin levels in the body. It's just perfect for one of those "I really need something sweet" days.
Go for it, it's all guilt free.

Serves: 2
Ingredients:
- 8 dates, pitted
- Half cup ice
- 1 cup of coconut milk
- Half avocado (peeled and pitted)
- 1 tablespoon coconut oil
- 1 teaspoon of cinnamon powder

Instructions:
1. Place all the above ingredients into the blender and mix/blend well.

Recipe #11 Veggie Freak

This is another super easy smoothie to help you add more veggies into our diet. Drinking veggies is much easier than eating them. And it takes less time for sure! Just set it, drink it and forget it.

I love to have this smoothie in the morning because it feels so good to cross it off my daily health goals list. Done!

Serves: 2
Ingredients:
- 1 cup leafy greens of your choice (it's a great way to use some of your left overs)
- 2 celery stalks, chopped
- Half cup broccoli florets, cooked chopped
- 1 cucumber, peeled and chopped
- 1 banana, peeled
- A few dates, pitted
- 1 cup coconut water
- Half cup ice

Instructions:
1. Place all the listed ingredients in a blender and mix/blend well.
2. Pour and enjoy.

Recipe #12 Creamy Dream Smoothie

This is an amazing smoothie recipe if you are craving something sweet and creamy. You can even freeze it and serve it as an ice cream!

Serves: 1
Ingredients:
- 1 avocado (peeled and pitted)
- 1 small banana, peeled
- 1 tablespoon chia seeds
- 1 teaspoon cinnamon powder
- 1 cup coconut milk
- Optional: paleo friendly cocoa ribs to garnish

Instructions:
1. Blend all except the ice for as long as possible.
2. Pulse in ice or skip the ice and freeze for ½ hour.
3. Serve in a dessert bowl and sprinkle over some cocoa ribs.
4. Enjoy!

Recipe #13 Mango Protein Smoothie

This smoothie just perfect for breakfast or as a quick snack. It is very high in protein and good fats and will help you prevent sugar cravings.

Serves: 2

Ingredients:
- 1 frozen mango, chopped
- A handful of soaked almonds
- 1 tablespoon powdered chia seeds
- 2 cups almond milk
- 1 cup arugula leaves, washed
- Half avocado, peeled, pitted
- Handful of blueberries

Instructions:
1. Blend all in a blender.
2. Enjoy!

Recipe #14 Easy Tropical Smoothie

This amazing and naturally sweet tropical smoothie is very clever in its design as it also sneaks in some greens and ginger.
Ginger really spices it up and is a great ingredient to add to your smoothies to prevent colds and inflammation.

Serves: 2
Ingredients:
- half cup spinach
- half cup guava
- 1-inch ginger
- half cup papaya, chopped
- 1 cup coconut water
- Ice, as needed

Instructions:
1. Place all the above ingredients in a blender. Carefully mix to attain the desired consistency.
2. Pulse in ice.
3. Enjoy!

Recipe #15 Cucumber Paleo Soup Smoothie

This smoothie can also be served as a soup. And you can easily make it in just a few minutes.

If you want to serve it as a soup, I recommend you add in some hard-boiled eggs, jam, bacon or smoked salmon. I also like to throw in some olives or other raw veggies.

Enjoy!

Serves: 1
Ingredients:
- 2 cucumbers, peeled
- 1 celery stalk
- 1 avocado (peeled and pitted)
- A handful of fresh cilantro
- 1 cup filtered water
- Pinch of Himalaya salt
- Pinch of black pepper
- Juice of half a lemon to taste

Instructions:
1. Blend all and enjoy!
2. Serve as a smoothie or as a soup.

Recipe #16 Paleo Zucchini Dream

Zucchini is one of the best alkaline paleo super foods. It's high in minerals and vitamins and low in calories. It blends really well with other greens as well as all kind of fruits.

Serves: 1-2
Ingredients:
- 1 zucchini, peeled
- Half green apple, peeled
- Half teaspoon cinnamon
- A few kale leaves
- 1 cup coconut water
- ½ cup ice

Instructions:
1. Blend all ingredients.
2. Pulse ice and enjoy!

Recipe #17 Watermelon Hydration

Watermelon is rich in the amino acid called citrulline and is useful in muscle recovery. It blends really well with greens and gives your smoothie a nice, refreshing taste too.

Serves: 2
Ingredients:
- 1 cup chopped watermelon
- 1 cup blueberries (fresh or frozen)
- A few broccoli florets, cooked
- Half cup spinach
- 1 cup coconut water
- 1 teaspoon maca powder
- Half cup ice (you can omit if using frozen blueberries)

Instructions:
1. Put all in a blender and mix to desired consistency.
2. Enjoy!

Recipe #18 Mediterranean Gazpacho Smoothness

Gazpacho is a traditional Spanish vegetable smoothie-like soup. It can be served both as a soup as well as a smoothie. It's one of my favorite lunch-time Paleo smoothies. It's very easy to make and you can serve it with some leftovers like meat, fish or hard-boiled eggs. That allows a perfectly balanced diet, full of greens, fresh veggies and full of protein to help you stay full for hours.

Serves: 2

Ingredients:
- 1 green onion, sliced
- 2 tablespoon fresh lemon juice
- A handful of chopped celery
- 1 cucumber, peeled and chopped
- 1 carrot, peeled and chopped
- 8 big, peeled, diced and seeded tomatoes
- 1 cup almond, dairy-free yogurt (you can also use coconut yoghurt)
- 1 teaspoon ground black pepper
- 1 tablespoon extra-virgin olive oil
- 1 small clove of garlic
- Himalaya salt to taste
- 8 fresh basil leaves to garnish

Instructions:
1. Put all ingredients in blender and mix well.
2. If needed, add some water and blend again.
3. Allow the gazpacho to cool.
4. Serve chilled in a bowl, decorated with basil leaves. Enjoy!

Recipe #19 Celery Veggie Snack

This is a super healing and weight loss stimulating green paleo smoothie.

Mint is very refreshing and relaxing. It also makes this smoothie taste amazing!

Serves: 1

Ingredients:
- 1 small cucumber, peeled and chopped
- Handful of spinach
- 1 grapefruit, peeled
- 1 cup coconut milk
- Half cup ice
- 3 mint leaves
- Optional: a bit of thick coconut milk for a creamy consistency

Instructions:
1. Place the above ingredients in your blender and process until smooth.
2. Enjoy!

Recipe #20 Kale Weight Loss Magician

Kale is a fabulous for weight loss. It is rich in fiber, phytonutrients, as well as tons of vitamins and minerals.

It blends really well with apples and other weight loss stimulating ingredients such as cinnamon and mint.

Serves: 1
Ingredients:
- 1 cup kale leaves, washed and chopped
- 1 teaspoon spirulina powder
- 1 cup almond or coconut milk
- 1 tablespoon coconut oil
- 2 green apples
- Handful of fresh mint leaves
- 1 teaspoon cinnamon powder
- Half lime, peeled

Instructions:
1. Mix all in a blender.
2. Pour into your cup and enjoy!

Recipe #21 Easy Tahini Smoothie

This smoothie uses tahini which makes it a nice, creamy and super filling smoothie. It's perfect for a quick breakfast or as a snack.

Serves: 1-2
Ingredients:
- 1 cup fresh blueberries
- A handful of leafy greens if your choice
- 1 big red apple, peeled
- 1 cup almond milk
- 2 tablespoons of Tahini
- Optional: maple syrup, a few dates or stevia to sweeten, if needed

Instructions:
1. Using a blender, mix all the above ingredients together.
2. Enjoy!

Recipe #22 Full Brain Power

I found this smoothie very helpful for long writing sessions or whenever I need to focus. Oh, and it tastes delicious too.

Another super healthy and guilt free smoothie. Whenever you feel like grabbing some chocolate, grab this smoothie instead!

Serves: 1-2

Ingredients:
- 1 cup coconut milk
- A few dates, pitted
- 1 orange, peeled
- 3 tablespoons organic cocoa powder
- 1 teaspoon maca powder
- 1 teaspoon cinnamon powder
- 1 tablespoon chia seed powder (or chia seeds)

Instructions:
1. Place all the ingredients in a blender.
2. Process until smooth, serve and enjoy!

Recipe #23 Good Carbs Smoothie

This smoothie is perfect for an active lifestyle. It offers good carbs, protein and fats to keep you going for hours!

Serves: 1

Ingredients:

- 1 cup unsweetened almond or coconut milk
- Half cup frozen strawberries
- A handful of cashew nuts
- 1-inch fresh ginger, peeled
- Pinch of cinnamon powder
- Half cup smashed pumpkin

Instructions:

1. Put all ingredients in a blender and mix well.
2. Add ginger
3. Enjoy!

Recipe #24 Green Date Smoothie

If you don't like the idea of eating green salads all the time, this smoothie offers an amazing alternative. You can mix your greens with some naturally sweet fruits and paleo approved superfoods to help you thrive!

Serves: 2
Ingredients:
- 1 cup kale, fresh
- 2 cups coconut milk
- Half cup pineapple, chopped
- 1 big kiwi, peeled
- 1 orange, peeled
- 1 teaspoon cinnamon powder
- A few fresh dates, pitted

Instructions:
1. Place all the other ingredients in a blender.
2. Blend and enjoy!

Recipe #25 Easy Berry Best

This smoothie combines natural fiber and vitamin C from fresh fruits with an immune system boosting properties of honey and the healing properties of the green, alkaline superfood chlorella.
To your health!

Serves: 3
Ingredients:
- 1 cup of coconut milk
- 1 cup fresh blueberries
- A few slices of banana
- A few slices of orange
- 1 teaspoon chlorella powder
- A dash of honey
- Ice cubes

Instructions:
1. Blend all the ingredients in a food processor.
2. Pour in a glass and enjoy!

Recipe #26 Watermelon Refreshment

Not only is this smoothie super hydrating and refreshing, but it's also super filling and will help you stay energized for hours.

Serves: 2-3
Ingredients:
- 1 cup of watermelon, cubed, seeded and chilled
- Half banana, peeled
- 1 small avocado, peeled and pitted
- A few slices of lemon
- 1 cup water, filtered
- Ice cubes (optional)

Instructions:
1. Blend until thoroughly combined and smooth.
2. If needed, toss in some ice cubes and enjoy.

Recipe #27 Papaya Weight Loss Smoothie Tea

Papaya is one of the best fruits to enjoy while trying to lose weight. It can also effectively help reduce bloating and other digestive problems. This smoothie also uses red tea and green tea.
Both red and green teas are mild stimulants and are very well known for their fat burn properties.

Serves: 2-3

Ingredients:
- 1 small papaya, peeled, seeded and cubed
- 1 teaspoon cinnamon powder
- A few slices of pineapple
- 1 cup water
- 1 green tea bag (or 1 teaspoon of green tea)
- 1 red tea bag (or 1 teaspoon of red tea)

Instructions:
1. Boil 1 cup of water.
2. Add in the green and red tea and leave to cool down a bit.
3. When cooled down, in a blender, combine the tea with papaya, pineapple and cinnamon.
4. Process well until smooth.
5. Enjoy!

Recipe #28 Creamy Balancer

This creamy smoothie is awesome for hot summer days. It's full of superfoods too. For example, maca powder helps re-balance hormones and Ashwagandha is an ancient Ayurvedic herb that helps sooth anxiety.

Serves: 1-2
Ingredients:
- 1 cup almond milk
- Half cup chamomile tea, cooled down
- 1 banana, peeled and pitted
- 1 orange, peeled
- Half teaspoon maca powder
- Half teaspoon Ashwagandha powder
- 1-inch ginger, peeled
- 1 teaspoon lemon juice, fresh
- Some ice cubes

Instructions:
1. Place all the ingredients in a blender.
2. Blend until creamy and smooth.
3. Drop in ice cubes and enjoy the creamy smoothie chilled.

To learn more about Ashwagandha I recommend you read my book: ***Ayurveda: ASHWAGANDHA: The Miraculous Herb! -Holistic Solutions & Proven Healing Recipes for Health, Beauty, Weight Loss & Hormone Balance***

Recipe #29 Vitamin C Delight

This recipe uses grapefruit and green tea. These are very helpful in weight loss and will help you stay energized and hydrated.

Serves: 1-2
Ingredients:
- 1 whole orange, peeled and sliced
- 1 whole grapefruit, peeled and sliced
- 1 cup green tea, cooled down
- A few slices of banana
- Half cup coconut water or coconut milk

Instructions:
1. Place all the ingredients in a blender.
2. Process until smooth.
3. Drop a few ice cubes in the glass and serve right away.

Recipe #30 Creamy Spinach Beauty Smoothie

This smoothie is not a typical fruity smoothie. It's actually spicy and can even be served as a soup (warm or chilled, whatever you prefer). It's very easy to digest and full of greens and vital nutrients which makes it perfect for detox days or whenever you feel like you need more energy.

Serves: 1
Ingredients:
- 1 cup of fresh spinach leaves, washed
- 1 whole avocado, pitted, peeled and diced
- 1 teaspoon of fresh lime juice
- 1 cup of almond milk
- A handful of cashews, unsalted (soak in filtered water for a few hours)
- Black pepper and Himalaya salt to taste
- Fresh cilantro leaves to garnish
- Optional: 2 small chili flakes if you like it spicy
- Optional: black pepper to taste

Instructions:
1. Blend all the ingredients until smooth.
2. Serve as a quick snack smoothie or as a soup.
3. (if you serve it as a soup, you can add in some hard-boiled eggs, fish, meat or nuts)

Recipe 31 Green Refreshment

This smoothie makes drinking greens not only painless but actually fun. Balance is the key. Focus on the ingredients you like and then make it your goal to add in some greens here and there. It will make an incredible difference in your wellbeing.

Serves: 1-2
Ingredients:
- Half cup fresh cherries, pitted
- Half cup fresh blueberries
- 1 green apple
- 1 tablespoon of any paleo-friendly protein powder of your choice, or chia seed powder
- A handful of spinach leaves, washed
- 1 cup of chilled coconut milk

Instructions:
1. Place all the ingredients in a blender.
2. Process until smooth.
3. Serve chilled with ice cubes and fresh mint leaves.
4. Enjoy!

Recipe #32 Beautiful Skin Smoothie

This smoothie combines the best of anti-age ingredients that are inexpensive and accessible. What more can you want?
Plus, it tastes delicious and is very inexpensive to make.

Serves: 1-2
Ingredients:
- 4 big tomatoes, peeled
- 1 lemon, peeled
- 2 carrots, peeled
- 1 grapefruit, peeled
- 1-inch ginger, peeled
- 1 cup of water, filtered

Instructions:
1. Blend all the ingredients.
2. Serve and enjoy!

Recipe #33 Creamy Paleo Protein Smoothie

This smoothie offers the best of plant-based Paleo. After all, Paleo is not only about eating meat. It's all about balance and creating a variety of meals that help you stay energized.

Serves: 1-2
Ingredients:
- 1 banana, peeled
- 1 orange, peeled
- A handful of walnuts, soaked for a few hours
- A handful of hazelnuts, soaked for a few hours
- 1 cup hazelnut milk
- 1 teaspoon nutmeg powder
- 1 teaspoon cinnamon powder

Instructions:
1. Blend all the ingredients.
2. Serve and enjoy.

Recipe #34 Ginger Mystery Smoothie

Ginger adds to anti-inflammatory properties of your smoothies and it really tastes amazing. You can also experiment by adding some honey if you like sweet smoothies.
Enjoy!

Serves: 1
Ingredients:
- 2 pears, peeled
- 1 cup almond milk
- 1 banana, peeled
- 1-inch ginger, peeled
- 1 teaspoon spirulina

Instructions:
1. Blend the apple and banana slices with coconut milk.
2. Add the peach and crushed ginger.
3. Drop in a few ice cubes, serve and enjoy.

Recipe #35 Tasty Veggie Smoothie

This is another simple veggie smoothie that can also be served as a soup.

Servings: 2
Ingredients:
- 2 big carrots, peeled and chopped
- 3 celery stalks, chopped
- A couple dashes of habanero hot sauce
- 2 big cucumbers, peeled and chopped
- 1 cup water
- 1 cup cashew milk (or coconut milk)
- a drizzle of avocado oil
- Himalaya salt to taste, if needed

Instructions:
1. Place through a blender.
2. Process until smooth.
3. Enjoy!

Recipe #36 Spicy Spinach Smoothie

Spinach blends really well with sweet apples. Adding some ginger, cinnamon and turmeric not only helps spice it up, but it also helps beat inflammation.

Chia seeds are one of the best plant-based sources of protein and it's always good to add some to your smoothies.

Serves: 2
Ingredients:
- 1 cup of fresh spinach
- 2 big red apples, peeled
- 1-inch ginger, peeled
- 1-inch turmeric root, peeled
- 1 cup fresh carrot or beetroot juice
- 1 tablespoon avocado oil
- Half teaspoon cinnamon
- 2 tablespoons chia seeds

Instructions:
1. Place all the ingredients through a juicer.
2. Extract the juice, pour it in a big glass.
3. Add in some melted coconut oil.
4. Stir well and enjoy.

Recipe #37 Easy Antioxidant Smoothie

This smoothie is great as a quick, light morning smoothie to help you eliminate toxins. It's also fantastic as a refreshing summer drink.

Servings: 2
Ingredients:
- 1 cup of watermelon, chopped
- 1 lemon, peeled
- 1 lime, peeled
- 1 cup water, filtered
- Honey, to sweeten, if needed
- Optional: ice cubes

Instructions:
1. Place all the ingredients in a blender.
2. Process until smooth, serve and enjoy!

Recipe #38 Simple Apple Lemon Juice

Apples help maintain a healthy digestive system.
They are full of fiber and will help you stay full for many hours.
In this smoothie, they combine very well with oranges and arugula leaves.

Servings: 2
Ingredients:
- 2 apples, peeled and chopped
- 2 oranges, peeled and halved
- 1 cup arugula leaves
- Half teaspoon maca
- 1 cup water, filtered
- Half cup thick coconut milk, or cashew milk

Instructions:
1. Place all the ingredients in a blender.
2. Process until smooth and enjoy!

Recipe #39 Honeydew Melon Green Juice

This is a super hydrating smoothie that combines the healing power of greens and fruits.

Romaine lettuce and cucumbers are great "beginner" veggies as their taste is very mild.

Servings: 2
Ingredients:
- 4 medium cucumbers, peeled and chopped
- 1 cup of honeydew melon
- 4 half cup romaine lettuce
- 2 apples, peeled
- 1 cup coconut water

Instructions:
1. Place all the ingredients in a blender.
2. Process until smooth.
3. Enjoy!

Recipe #40 Easy Green Protein Smoothie

This smoothie combines spirulina powder with chia seeds, almonds and leafy greens which makes it a great, energy boosting green protein smoothie.

Servings: 2-3
Ingredients:
- 2 green bell peppers, chopped
- Half cup kale leaves, washed
- 1 inch of ginger, peeled
- Half teaspoon spirulina powder
- 1 teaspoon chia seeds
- A handful of almonds, soaked
- 2 cups almond milk
- 2 slices of lime, to garnish
- Fresh ice cubes

Instructions:
1. Place all the ingredients (except lime) in a blender
2. Process until smooth.
3. Pour in a glass, add in some ice cubes.
4. Garnish with lime slices.
5. Serve and enjoy!

Recipe #41 Green Coconut Smoothie

This smoothie is a perfect detox smoothie to enjoy first thing in the morning. Coconut water can be replaced with "normal", filtered water, or fennel tea infusion.

Servings: 2
Ingredients:
- 1 cup kale, chopped
- 1 green apple, peeled, and cut into smaller pieces
- 1 cup of coconut water
- 2 lemons, peeled
- Optional: honey to sweeten

Instructions:
1. Place all the ingredients in a blender.
2. Process until smooth.
3. Enjoy!

Recipe #42 Hidden Broccoli Smoothie

This smoothie is a great recipe to "recycle" some broccoli leftovers. Broccoli, just like all kinds of green veggies as well as leafy greens, blends really well with oranges.

Servings: 2
Ingredients:
- 1 cup cooked broccoli, chopped
- 2 oranges, peeled and cut into smaller pieces
- 1 cup coconut milk
- 1 teaspoon cinnamon powder

Instructions:
1. Blend all the ingredients.
2. Pour into a glass and enjoy!

Recipe #43 Green Tea Fat Burn Smoothie

This recipe uses green tea to help you boost your energy levels and burn fat. At the same time, it offers a blend of highly alkalizing fruits and veggies combined with ginger to reduce inflammation.

Parsley gives this smoothie a really original taste while adding lots of nutrients and Vitamin A.

Servings: 2
Ingredients:
- 2 grapefruits, peeled and cut into smaller pieces
- 2 cucumbers, peeled and cut into smaller pieces
- 1-inch ginger, peeled
- A handful of parsley
- 1 cup green tea, cooled down
- Optional: honey to sweeten, if needed.

Instructions:
1. Blend all the ingredients using a blender or a food processor.
2. Pour into a glass or a bowl.
3. Enjoy!

Recipe #44 Healthy Glow Smoothie

This smoothie is one of the best, natural recipes, you can try to have that "healthy glow" around you and take care of your skin.

Servings: 2
Ingredients:
- 4 carrots, peeled and chopped
- 2 oranges, peeled and cut into smaller pieces
- 1 grapefruit, peeled and cut into smaller pieces
- Half cup parsley
- 1 cup organic tomato juice
- 2-inch turmeric, peeled
- A few ice cubes (optional)
- A dash of cinnamon powder (optional)

Instructions:
1. Place all the ingredients through a blender.
2. Process well until smooth.
3. Drink to your health and natural beauty!
4. Enjoy!

Recipe #45 Antioxidant Veggie Smoothie

Even though tomatoes are very often called "a veggie" (even I admit to discriminating against it by indirectly calling it a "veggie" by writing the title of this recipe), it's actually a fruit.

And it's a great ingredient to make a delicious, spicy smoothie that can be also served as a soup.

Servings: 2
Ingredients:
- 4 tomatoes, peeled and cut into smaller pieces
- Handful of parsley
- 1 tablespoon chia seed powder
- 1 Garlic clove, peeled
- 1-inch ginger, peeled
- Himalaya salt to taste

Instructions:
1. Place all the ingredients through a blender.
2. Process well until smooth.
3. Enjoy!

Recipe #46 Easy Beet Smoothie

Beets and carrots are miraculous veggies. Full of fiber, vitamins and minerals they can be easily turned into a delicious, natural sweet smoothie that can also be turned into a soup.

Servings: 2
Ingredients:
- 3 medium carrots, peeled and cut into smaller pieces
- 5 small beets, peeled
- half bunch parsley (optional)
- 1 cup coconut water, or filtered water

Instructions:
1. Place all the ingredients in a blender.
2. Blend well until smooth.
3. Enjoy!

Recipe #47 Simple Nutrition Smoothie

This smoothie is very easy to make and the ingredients are easily accessible. Carrots and apples blend very well and offer an amazing sweet taste that makes you crave more and more of it.
Cinnamon takes that taste to the next level.

Servings: 2-3
Ingredients:
- 4 green apples, peeled, chopped
- 4 carrots, peeled
- 2 cups of almond milk
- 2 tablespoons chia seeds

Instructions:
1. Blend all the ingredients.
2. Pour into a glass and enjoy.

Recipe #48 Arugula Power Olive Smoothie

I am a big fan of arugula and I love adding it to my salads. But, arugula leaves are also great for smoothies. Most people fear green and veggie smoothies because they are not aware how tasty they can actually be. Like I always say.

Drinking your veggies is much easier than eating them. And it tastes less time and effort too.

Oh and this smoothie can also be served as a dip or a soup.

Servings: 2
Ingredients:
- 1 cup arugula leaves
- 1 big avocado, peeled and pitted
- Half cup black olives, pitted
- Half cup green olives, pitted
- 2 big tomatoes, peeled
- Half cup water, filtered
- Himalaya salt to taste
- Black pepper to taste
- Optional: chili powder if you like it spicy

Instructions:
1. Place all the ingredients in a blender.
2. Process until smooth, serve and enjoy!

Recipe #49 Tantalizing Green Smoothie Soup

Once again, we are making a super tasty green veggie smoothie that can also be served as a dip, appetizer, or even a warm soup. To your health, enjoy!

Servings: 2
Ingredients:
- 1 cup green olives, pitted
- Half cup fresh parsley leaves
- 2 cucumbers, peeled
- Half avocado, peeled and pitted
- 1 cup coconut or almond milk (unsweetened)
- Himalaya salt and black pepper to taste

Instructions:
1. Place all the ingredients in a blender.
2. Process until smooth and enjoy!

Recipe #50 Re-Balancing Carrot Smoothie

Carrots will help you stay hydrated and reduce unwanted sugar cravings for hours. Ashwagandha powder is a natural herb to help you re-gain balance and fight off stress.

Servings: 2
Ingredients:
- 4 carrots, peeled and chopped
- a pinch of Ashwagandha powder
- 1 teaspoon cinnamon powder
- 1 cup of thick coconut milk

Instructions:
1. Blend all the ingredients using a blender or a food processor.
2. Pour into a glass and enjoy!

Recipe #51 Easy Almond Butter & Banana Smoothie

Bananas are high in potassium, vitamin B6 and Vitamin C, while the almond butter is an excellent source of protein. The bananas are best used frozen and I find the best way to freeze them for easy use is to cut them up into small slices, then spread them out on an oven tray with a sheet of baking paper on top.

This way they will be easy to grab from the freezer and throw in the blender when you're ready to go!

Serves: 1-2

Ingredients:

- 2 bananas, sliced
- half teaspoon spirulina powder
- 2 tablespoons almond butter
- A handful of spinach
- 1 cup of almond milk

Instructions:

1. Place all ingredients in a blender.
2. Blend until smooth.
3. Serve in a chilled glass and enjoy!

Recipe #52 Sexy Flaxseed Smoothie

The flaxseed meal is paleo friendly and also an excellent source of Omega-3 fatty acids, aka 'good fats'. Good fats are also found in almonds, so this smoothie is packed full of both healthy fats and protein.

After having this smoothie, not only will you feel full and satisfied but you will also get an energy boost from bananas and natural source of protein.

Serves: 2-3

Ingredients:

- 2 bananas, sliced
- a handful of almonds, soaked
- a few kale leaves, chopped
- 1 big peach, peeled
- 1 cup of almond milk,
- 2 tablespoons of flaxseed meal

Instructions:

1. Place all ingredients in a blender.

2. Blend until combined and almonds are blitzed.

3. Serve into a chilled glass and enjoy!

Recipe #53 Blueberry Optimal Protein Smoothie

This blueberry breakfast smoothie is the perfect way to start your morning. It can be used as a meal replacement for your normal breakfast, as the ingredients used will provide you with enough nutrients and energy to keep you active and alert all day. If you're in a rush, sleep in or aren't usually a breakfast eater – then this smoothie will change your life!

It's easy to prepare and will keep you going all day. It provides a great slow release of energy from the cashews, antioxidants and essential nutrients from the blueberries. It's thick, delicious and will make you feel full until your next meal. Oats are not paleo, so this smoothie is a great, paleo friendly alternative because it uses cashews instead. It makes this smoothie taste super creamy and irresistible.

Serves: 3-4

Ingredients:

- 1 cup of almond milk
- half cup of fresh blueberries
- handfuls of raw cashews, unsalted
- 1 teaspoon of vanilla extract
- 1 tablespoon of hemp seeds
- 1 tablespoon of chia seeds

Instructions:

1. Blend all the ingredients using a blender or a food processor.
2. Enjoy!

Recipe #54 Mango & Almond Butter Smoothie

It's no secret by now that nut butters are paleo friendly and an excellent source of protein. Almond butter is high in protein, low in saturated fat and has a great taste. The almond butter gives this smoothie a thick, creamy texture making it taste amazing and is very filling. Mangoes are also a fantastic source of important vitamins that will help you stay energized and alert.

Serves: 4

Ingredients:

- 2 cups of mango, cut into chunks
- 8 tablespoons of almond butter
- Half cup of almond milk
- a few dates, pitted
- 1 lime, peeled
- A dash of water
- A few mint leaves
- Optional: honey to taste

Instructions:

1. Place all the ingredients in a blender.
2. Blend together until well combined.
3. If needed, add a dash of water to thin the mixture.
4. Pour into a chilled glass, garnish with some mint leaves and serve.

DELICIOUS PALEO SMOOTHIE RECIPES

Recipe #55 Cinnamon Protein Smoothie

This is an incredibly delicious smoothie that can be used as a breakfast replacement if you are on the go. Cinnamon & apple is a classic flavor combination and when combined in this smoothie provides a great source of protein and vitamins. The main source of protein from this smoothie is from the nuts and the almond butter.

Serves: 2-3

Ingredients:

- 2 apples, sliced
- half cup almonds, soaked overnight
- half teaspoon of cinnamon
- 1 tablespoon of almond butter
- half cup of almond milk
- A dash of water

Instructions:

1. Add the almond milk and almonds to a high-powered blender.

2. Blend until well combined. Allow to rest for 2-3 minutes.

3. Add the rest of the ingredients to the blender and blitz until well combined.

4. Pour into a chilled smoothie glass and enjoy!

DELICIOUS PALEO SMOOTHIE RECIPES

Recipe #56 Spinach & Avocado Smoothie

This savory smoothie recipe packs its secret punch of protein from hulled hemp seeds. Hulled hemp seeds can be purchased in the healthy foods section of your local super market and are an incredible natural source of protein. Spinach is also a great all-rounder in smoothie recipes, blends easy, proteins an extra bit of protein and doesn't affect the flavor of the beverage at all.

Serves: 2

Ingredients:

- 2 tablespoons hemp seeds
- 1 cup coconut milk
- 1 cup spinach leaves
- half avocado, peeled and pitted
- 2 large pitted dates

Instructions:

1. Add all ingredients to a blender.
2. Process until well combined.
3. Pour into a glass, serve and enjoy!

Recipe #57 The Green Machine Protein Smoothie

Spinach in packed full of iron (more than you will find in a T-bone steak) and has also been found to work as an appetite suppressant. If you drink this smoothie first thing in the morning, chances are you'll feel full for longer and it will help you lose weight!

Serves: 2

Ingredients:

- 1 cup spinach
- 1 cup cucumber, chopped
- Half cup of celery, chopped
- Half cup of fresh watercress
- 1 chard leaf
- 1 cup coconut or cashew milk
- A handful of cilantro leaves
- Himalaya salt to taste

Instructions:

1. Add all ingredients to a high-powered blender and blitz until well combined.
2. Serve and enjoy!

Recipe #57 Goji Berry Dream Smoothie

Goji berries contain a great number of antioxidants that help to give you healthy skin and protect the eyes. They also help to boost your immune system.

At the same time, they provide a source of complex carbohydrates which will ensure you have a sustained release of energy, helping you to keep active throughout the entire day.

Serves: 2

Ingredients:

- 2 cups almond milk
- 1 banana
- 2 tablespoons of cacao nibs
- 1 teaspoon of maca powder
- 2 teaspoons of flaxseed meal
- 1 tablespoon of chia seeds
- 1 teaspoon of hemp seeds
- 1 teaspoon of vanilla extract
- A small handful of goji berries, to garnish

Instructions:

1.Add all the ingredients into a high-powered blender.

2.Blitz until well combined.

3.Pour into a chilled glass.

4.Sprinkle Goji Berries or other fruits on top and serve.

Recipe #58 Paleo Chocolate Smoothie

This chocolate and strawberry flavored smoothie not only tastes amazing, but it provides a huge range of health benefits thanks to the superfoods that are included in the recipe.

Strawberries have a huge range of healthy nutrients and vitamins including magnesium, phosphorus, potassium, iodine, folate, dietary fiber, vitamin B6, biotin and omega-3 fatty acids.

Serves: 2

Ingredients:

- 2 cups of almond milk
- 1 cup of strawberries
- Half cup blueberries
- 1 tablespoon of cacao nibs
- 1 tablespoon of hemp seeds
- 1 tablespoon of chia seeds
- A small handful of raw almonds

Instructions:

1. Add all ingredients into a high-powered blender.
2. Blend well.
3. Pour into a chilled glass and serve.

Recipe # 59 Chia Coconut Smoothie

Coconuts are an excellent source of B vitamins, as well as A & E, iron, magnesium, calcium and sodium.

Chia seeds will give you a boost of energy and provide you with essential omega-3 fatty acids, while the protein source will be provided by the cashews.

Serves: 2-3

Ingredients:

- 2 cups of cashew milk
- 4 tablespoons desiccated coconut
- 1 small banana
- 2 tablespoons chia seeds
- a handful of raw cashews

Instructions:

1. Place all the ingredients in a blender.
2. Process well until smooth.
3. Enjoy!

Recipe #60 Pumpkin Seed Protein Smoothie

But if it is a hot day and you are looking for a delicious smoothie that isn't too filling but will cool you down, then pumpkin seeds are a great source of natural high protein.

Serves: 1-2

Ingredients:

- 1 cup of coconut milk
- 1 cup of watermelon, cut into chunks
- 2 tablespoons of pumpkin seeds
- 1 tablespoon avocado oil

Instructions:

1. Add all ingredients to a blender.
2. Process until well combined.
3. Pour into a chilled glass and serve.

DELICIOUS PALEO SMOOTHIE RECIPES

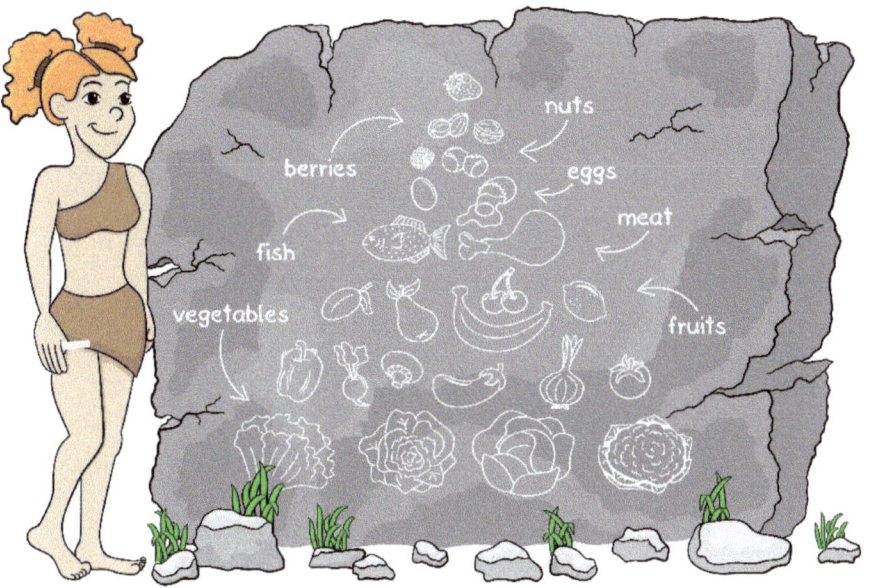

Final Words and Your Paleo Quick Start Guide

We hope you enjoyed the recipes and feel inspired to live a Paleo lifestyle.

We are adding this short Paleo guide to help you on your health journey.

Remember, it's not about being perfect. Even if you do Paleo "part time", but you listen to your body and focus on adding as many healthy foods as possible, you are good to go.

It's not about going hungry or getting too caught up in counting calories.

Paleo Lifestyle Made Easy

The Paleo diet is an approach to eating that originated a long time ago, during the Paleolithic era. This time frame started about 2.5 million years ago and ended around 10,000 years before our time. It avoids eating foods that only became part of the human diet after the agricultural revolution.

The idea is that diseases like cancer and diabetes started around the same time that we began growing our own foods. The underlying principle is that the hunter-gatherers' diet is the reason they did not develop such diseases.

While we cannot be sure that their diet is what kept them healthy, there is enough research that concludes that foods banned from

Paleo diets have little or no beneficial nutritional value. They have also been proven to interrupt normal hormonal balances, cause inflammation, and damage the lining of the gut. Eating Paleo will help to balance our bodies internally, protect the kidneys, protect the digestive tract from destructive proteins like gluten, and keep the liver and pancreas from having to work too hard.

Many names and titles have been given to this age-old eating program: the Paleolithic diet, Paleolithic nutrition, Paleo diet, Stone Age diet, caveman diet, and hunter-gatherer diet. Paleo Diet is an effort to go back to eating how we were biologically intended to eat. This method enables us to fuel our bodies properly so that they may function at their full genetic potential and start living healthier immediately. Foods that could be collected and consumed by hunting and gathering are what need to focus on. Primal eating at its best.

For me, I like to think of it as a Paleo perspective, not an actual diet. It could also be called a template. However you look at it, it is a lifestyle change. The goal is to eat like our ancestors did millions of years ago before the Agricultural Revolution.

Here are seven guidelines for Paleo nutrition that helped me to get a better idea of the principles involved in this primal nutritional practice.

1. **Increase protein intake.**

15% of the calories in most diets are from protein. When adhering to Paleo, that percentage must be much higher. It should be between 19-35 percent. A large amount of animal protein is required.

2. **Decrease carbohydrate intake and eat foods lower on the glycemic index.**

Most of the carbs will come from vegetables (and a few fruits). They should take up between 35-45 percent of your daily caloric intake. Most of the foods you will eat will be low on the glycemic index. They will not make your blood sugar spike because they are assimilated slowly.

3. **Increase fiber consumption.**

Paleos get their fiber from non-starchy vegetables. Vegetables such as these usually contain a fiber content around 30 percent higher than processed grain and about eight times higher than whole grain. Even fruits have more fiber than whole and refined grains.

4. **Increase fat intake by eating more monounsaturated and polyunsaturated fats.**

You need to do this in combination with a good balance of Omega-3 and Omega-6 fats. It is a common misconception that health is related to how *much* fat you eat, when the *type* of fat you eat affects your health more. Increase monounsaturated and Omega-3 fats and remove Trans and Omega-6 polyunsaturated fats.

5. **Raise potassium while lowering sodium.**

Paleolithic humans consumed foods that were unrefined and fresh. Potassium levels in fresh foods are between 5-10 percent higher than sodium levels. Potassium helps the heart, kidneys, and other organs function correctly. People who have low potassium levels are more susceptible to elevated blood pressure, stroke, and cardiovascular disease. Excessive sodium levels can also cause the same problems. Many modern diets contain two times as much sodium as potassium.

6. Eat more alkaline than acidic foods.

When we consume food, it has either an acid or alkaline effect on your body. Even on a Paleo diet, it is necessary to keep this in mind because meat and fish are both acid-forming foods. Alkaline-producing foods include most vegetables and fruits. Having an acidic system for a long time can lead to atrophy of the muscles and bone, elevated blood pressure, kidney stones, and can trigger things like asthma and allergies.

7. Increase the intake of vitamins, phytochemicals, minerals, and antioxidants.

Whole grains are a poor source of these things. The few minerals and vitamins that are actually in whole grains are not usually processed and absorbed properly by the body. They do not contain vitamin C, A, or B12. There truly is no substitute for grass-produced and free-range meat or organic vegetables and fruits.

What foods did the cavemen eat? What foods did they hunt, and what did they go out and gather? These are two key questions to keep in mind when deciding what to eat on the Paleo diet.

Basic categories of foods to consume when eating Paleo:

- Grass-produced meats
- Fish and seafood
- Eggs
- Fresh fruits and vegetables
- Seeds

- Healthful oils (olive, walnut, flaxseed, macadamia, avocado, or coconut)

The foods included on the Paleo diet are foods that our cave-dwelling ancestors would have access to on a regular basis. Basic categories of what NOT to eat when eating Paleo:
- Cereals and grains
- Potatoes
- Legumes
- Sugars
- Processed foods
- Salt
- Dairy
- Refined vegetable oil

(Examples of legumes are):
- Beans
- Peas
- Lentils
- Soy

Essentially, if a caveman could not have eaten it 10,000 years ago, you cannot eat it now. No consuming packaged foods at all. If it contains chemicals or ingredients that you cannot pronounce, then it is probably not Paleo.

Inflammation is the body's natural response to invaders. I already discussed this problem and how "leaky gut" will lead to weight gain. It may be more important to note that "leaky gut" will lead to major health issues because it causes chronic inflammation. Cancer, asthma, headaches, allergies, arthritis, auto-immune disorders, heart disease, diabetes, depression, Alzheimer's, and osteoporosis are all caused by chronic inflammation. The list goes on and on.

Why does inflammation cause so many problems? Inflammation is an immune system response. It is used by the body to battle intruders that are unidentified or already deemed harmful. Well, how could something good cause such a problem? Let me explain it this way. It is like leaving the heater turned up and the thermostat not working. It never turns off when the environment gets to a certain temperature. Yes, you wanted to warm up, but if it never turns off, it will get way too hot. It will negatively affect whatever is in the environment.

Converting to a Paleolithic nutritional lifestyle has allowed me to eat a diet that is void of inflammatory foods. Aside from healing "leaky gut," thus allowing the immune system to calm down, Paleo diets also reduce inflammation in many other ways. I have highlighted a few below:

> ➤ The diet is high in vitamin D. Vitamin D has been proven to aid in reducing inflammation.

> ➤ The diet is high in phytonutrients, many of which have anti-inflammatory effects.

> ➤ The immune system reacts to factors in the environment that it has been exposed to (pollen, bacteria, molds, etc.) with inflammation. The Paleo diet has the effect of making the immune system less prone to react to these factors and also makes it more effective because it is not over-loaded.

> The Paleo perspective adjusts the Omega-3/Omega-6 proportion to a beneficial ratio and makes it an effective agent in battling inflammatory illnesses. An Omega-3/6 imbalance can result from eating vegetable oils, grain products, and a deficiency of DHA and EPA from animal products.

Reading labels is a must-do for any Paleo dieter. For the most part, anything with a label is probably something you do not want to buy. If it does have a label, but you can't pronounce the ingredients, do not purchase it. Here are some things that I keep in mind when I grocery shop:

Best = Zero ingredients

Better = One ingredient

Ok = Two ingredients

Pushing my luck = Three ingredients

No way = Four+ ingredients

Key words to remember when shopping to stock a Paleo kitchen: Organic, grass-fed, pasture-raised, wild-caught, free-range, and raw.

I had to replace everything in my pantry with new ingredients that I would be using in Paleo recipes. I had previewed these new recipes, and if you are anything like me, these ingredients sounded strange. They are staples of the Paleo kitchen and will benefit you in preparing many delicious Paleo meals and snacks. This a list of items that are usually used in Paleo recipes:

- Blanched almond flour

- Coconut flour

- Almond meal

- Extra virgin coconut Oil

- Refined coconut oil

- Palm shortening

- Arrowroot powder/Tapioca starch

- Ground flax meal

- Coconut milk

- Creamed coconut

- Unsweetened coconut flakes

- Unsweetened shredded coconut

- Nuts: Whole almonds, pecan halves, walnut halves, macadamia nuts, hazelnuts, pistachios, cashews, Brazil nuts

- Almond Butter

- Raw/natural cocoa powder

- Honey

- Raw maple syrup

- Leavening/Spices: Baking soda, cream of tartar, allspice, cinnamon, salt, cloves, cardamom, ground ginger, nutmeg, vanilla extract, vanilla bean, lemon juice

We Need Your Help

One more thing, before you go, could you please do us a quick favor?

It would be great if you could leave us a short review on Amazon. Don't worry, it doesn't have to be long. One sentence is enough. Let others know your favorite recipes and who you think this book can help.

Your opinion is very important.

Thank You once again for your support!

Join Our VIP Readers' Newsletter to Boost Your Wellbeing

Would you like to be notified about our new health and wellness books?

How about receiving them at deeply discounted prices? And before anyone else?

What about awesome giveaways, amazing health tips and motivation?

If that is something you are interested in, please visit the link below to join our newsletter:

www.HolisticWellnessBooks.com/newsletter

It's 100% free + spam free and you can easily unsubscribe whenever you want (although 99.9% of our readers decide to stay signed up and they love the book discounts and inspiration they are getting). We promise we will only email you with valuable and relevant information.

More Books in the *Paleo – Healthy Lifestyle Series*

These books are available on Amazon in eBook, paperback and audiobook format.

You will find them by looking for *Elena Garcia* in your local Amazon store, or going to:

www.YourWellnessBooks.com

Thank you again for taking an interest in my work,
Have an amazing day,
Elena